Feel it! Ultimate Strength

Feel it! Ultimate Strength

In fitness for men and woman

Marcel le Roux

iUniverse, Inc.
Bloomington

Feel it! Ultimate Strength

iUniverse books may be ordered through booksellers or by contacting:

iUniverse
1663 Liberty Drive
Bloomington, IN 47403
www.iuniverse.com
1-800-Authors (1-800-288-4677)

ISBN: 978-1-4620-6379-6 (sc)
ISBN: 978-1-4620-6380-2 (ebk)

Printed in the United States of America

iUniverse rev. date: 11/03/2011

CONTENTS

FOREWORD

The book started after many years of failure to reach fitness and physical goals. Going to the gym and then stopping after a month or so with no real results, used to be the norm. The body I wanted can be seen around us in magazines and on television on a constant basis.

One of my most important lessons I learned throughout my new journey is the high capabilities of the body. Capabilities much higher than what I had intended for myself. Our success and achievement rate can be so much higher, hence the reason I share these fitness secrets. The power that exists in and around me when I work out today can be measured through results and energy levels on a much higher standard.

Physical training has truly become bliss.

I can see myself in around 90% of people in any given gym only a few years ago. I wish not to see any lack in others who are trying to improve their fitness, however, different levels of physical attainability do exist.

Maximum levels of energy and physicality is available to anyone who wants it.

My intention for the person that constantly joins the gym is to find that much needed energy levels, therefore obtaining physical results you can see in the least amount of effort possible. It is amazing how easy it can be to reach desired results when a few crucial steps are taken. Although days do exist when a person will feel drained, they should be few and far between. These laziness aspects that occur can be avoided and treated in very little effort when realization kicks in.

In this book I have included all the necessary steps for achieving goals which would seem like a massive task to the mind and body. Please don't skip any parts and make sure that all is understood before attempting. I've tried to make it as simple as possible. I can understand that some of these training techniques will be tough to accept for some individuals. I do however insist in following these steps for ultimate results.

Any body you can imagine yourself in, can be realized when you follow the recipe.

These tips will be life-transforming to other athletes that need to work on their strength in various different sports. Various training secrets will be revealed for you to be one step ahead of the game.

Chapter 1

NUTRITION

Up to 80% of any results achieved in fitness, in most people, comes due to a balance in they're eating programme. That includes adequate amounts of water. The fact is that results are achieved outside the gym or fitness area when muscles are repairing. What do you do outside the gym that is so important? You eat and sleep together with all the other aspects that come with "repairing".

To achieve optimum results you can feel and see as you progress from the one level of fitness to the next, is easily obtained with the least amount of mental and physical effort through finding a balance in nutrition. Now at first it may sound like you know what a healthy diet consists of, and yes you might have a good idea of what is needed to achieve the results you play over and over in your mind, but you are maybe just not following the recipe.

When you actually try these recommended daily nutritional values, a new high can be reached that is absolutely vital in the art of muscle and strength building, and as a result, weight loss. To follow the balance is already a huge mile stone reached in the sport of weight lifting and fitness. No one or no machine can measure your own capabilities, but you can learn to FEEL GREAT and I know THAT to be the most important lesson. You can in fact start right now. So one thing you can do right now is to start feeling great. There are however a few "tricks" to attaining these feelings.

It always comes down to what you consume over the weekend and during training days. You have to admit to yourself at some point, and believe me you will, that substances such as alcohol in large quantities are just not going to contribute in desired results. The best thing about finding these "new" highs in energy levels is that you actually cut down on bad habits habitually without much thinking involved in the process. I'll leave the entire decision making up to you of what and how much you should consume. It is important to grow into something rather than making all these "impossible" changes. Ease into it and it will seem like nothing at all.

There is of course vital steps that need to be taken that comes with reaching desired results. It would be wise to stick to an eating programme as much as possible until a certain energy level is reached, that of which you would not have considered normal from previous training sessions. I have included eating ideas and programmes in the latter part of the book. You can skip to chapter 7 if you would like to apply some of these ideas while you work your way through the book.

When these "new" energy levels hit, and I can assure you they will, bad habits will habitually fall away or decrease as you go along. These great feelings are right in the midst of you, IF you can only take the first step.

Optimum results are inevitable when you apply a great programme.

It has to be a-nothing-less than great feeling that drives you to be what you want to be, or drives you to feel the way you want to feel. To avoid the mind coming into play as far as games (provoking negative emotions) are concerned, and therefore influencing decision making, is vital. It can't be a chore. Strenuous exercise has to be enjoyable for those great feelings to prolong in the mind and body. If it isn't fun then why do it. How do you achieve those good feelings? Keep reading.

To reach a high that WILL drag you back for more and more is actually easily available for everyone to enjoy without illegal substances. Brilliant varieties of products are however available, and they could play a crucial role in reaching you're new easily attainable physique. The majority of us have these products available to us at our fingertips, depending on the country you live in. We'll delve into that a little later in the book.

So where do you find the right nutritional programme and what does it consist of? Well the answer is in this book and everywhere around all people who want it. If nutrition is rocket science to you, than now is the time to start learning. It is not only the things you learn within these pages, but also an ongoing learning and growing process that must be realized. As we move along, you will come to find that it is actually not that hard to understand at all.

When you take the cells that make up the body, you will find various different components that can only be found in foods and a few others sources. These components make you who you are and determine the way you feel.

You are what you eat!

When there is a lack of one of these components, a signal travels back to the mind telling you to stop with whatever exercise it is you are attempting at any given time. Fatigue will eventually set in and THAT needs to be avoided and treated.

When they say you need a slice of a certain bread a day, then my best advice would be to try and make that compulsory food sources in your diet. It is easy to understand when you realize that your body needs certain things for optimum energy levels. Food such as fruit and vegetables has lots of energy, rye bread has ample amounts of fibre, and good fat (unsaturated) can be attained from something like an avocado pear. Everyone has different tastes in food. So you have to mix it up as you go along to reach that balance.

NOTE; all the different foods need to be consumed to attain a balanced nutritional diet. This will contribute to reaching those energy levels necessary for optimum results.

When there is a small lack in a component that the body is craving for, multi vitamins can be taken which I consider to be very important in any diet. Take the recommended daily allowance for optimum results.

Chapter 7 will show the amounts of food that should be consumed by the average individual. If you can only get as close to the recommended daily allowance, then so much the better. You also have to understand that you're body will crave for more than the recommended daily allowance, because you will in essence, reach higher levels of demand in the following weeks to come. Please don't hesitate to eat.

You will need to be on top of your game for you to be able to keep up with the programme provided.

When your body screams out for nourishment, don't delay, give it what it needs or do your planning so you don't find yourself in those situations where you are essentially starving yourself.

Always allow for ample amounts of nutrition for you to be ready for next day's training.

Your muscles are recovering and needs food to grow and repair. We are "tearing" the muscle to make it stronger. "Tear and repair" is the motto for the next few months.

1GRAM OF CARBOHYDRATE PER KILOGRAM OF BODY WEIGHT

A Good amount of carbohydrate amount that should be allowed is 1g of carbohydrate per kilogram of bodyweight. Stick to that where you can and use it as indications on your carbohydrate consumption. The amount might however increase as exercising continues. Don't consume any less than the suggested amount. This is only an indicator for you to be able to find that balance.

There are all sorts of carbohydrate compounds, so stick to the ones you love. Vary the different kinds of foods. As far as the foods go that you don't appreciate, try to get to know them. Even try and prepare them in different recipes so appreciation can become the next level. I don't particularly like broccoli, but I know what it does for the body, so I steam it and sprinkle cheese on them.

Start by reading the back of packaging of products that contain a lot of ingredients that will make you feel lazy.

I can assure you that in order for you to sustain you're new found high, you will think twice before you buy many of the usual products. I can't stretch enough how important food is for your new training programme. It will be introduced a little later in the book.

The new found energy will be addictive and you will truly believe in nutrition and finding a balance when training resumes. The odd lazy product will enter the body because of years and years of past conditioning, still that sensation from eating that odd snack will not prolong.

What you know is more important than what you have been taught.

Saturated fats flourish in these so called snacks and should be avoided on training days. They can put you off from training or you might not have it in you (mentally) to complete a whole training session at FULL PACE. You will find that my training programs at the latter part of the book are very demanding and yet so satisfying when adequate nutritional values are included in your diet.

2 GRAMS OF PROTIEN PER KILOGRAM OF BODY WEIGHT.

I do insist on 2 grams of protein per kilogram of bodyweight when serious muscle building is practised. Please refrain from exceeding this amount until higher levels of strenuous exercise are being experienced.

Protein shakes with minimum amounts of carbohydrates, like whey products, will benefit you're muscle growth and will help in repairing and as a result play a massive role in energy levels desired.
Fish and chicken holds the healthiest and most important part of protein intake. Protein shakes provide a quick fix when meals are not taken.

MEALS TAKEN 2-3 HOURS APART

Whey protein together with a small fruit like an apple will get you through to the next 2 to 3 hours. To sustain the 2 to 3 hour rule is not easy if you don't want it to be easy. I can already hear lots of excuses. The fact of the matter is that you should always try and come as close to your target as possible by taking you're eating times seriously. 2 to 3 shakes a day each together with a fruit is perfect. Varieties of nuts work perfect as a snack.

NOTE; protein shakes can be left out when you're providing yourself with sufficient protein via meals, which will be more advantageous to your body. Stay away from

too many protein shakes. You're meals are the most important and the shake is only there as an extra.

NOTE; there is no such thing as "meal replacement". No shake can ever compare to a piece of fish and steamed vegetables.

CRAMPING CAN BE AVOIDED—EXTRA SALT ADDED TO THE DIET.

Sprinkles of salt on your meal once a day would quickly sort out any problems in cramping of muscles. Please, however, see a physician when cramping continues. Cramping may also occur when a balanced diet is not followed. A replacement of salt will be obvious due to the demanding levels attained in the gym. Cramping can occur as result and a lack of salt in the body and should be avoided and treated.

HEADACHES SHOULD NEVER BE EXPERIENCED

The same goes with headaches. You should never get them. Dehydration usually comes as a result and the only way to get rid of them would be to stack up on water. I've added a chapter on dehydration to show how important water can be for nutritional purposes and the overall functioning of the body alike. Your body will be screaming for water when training schedules are properly followed.

Dehydration should be well understood and therefore avoided as much as possible.

NOTE; you should NEVER have a dry throat on training days. Always carry a bottle of WATER (nothing else but water should be consumed) around while you're training.

Chapter 2

ROLE MODELS

The second part, depending on the individual mind, can be life transforming and could just be what many people need. That is the psychological part of attaining one's desired physical appearance.

THE RULE IS SIMPLE; if you're not going there in your head then you are not going there in reality.

Most people don't travel in the mind or they do the first part which is to visualize these physical attributes, and then don't continue to believe that these goals or desires can be achieved.

Results are inevitable in reaching fitness goals, if you believe in them and if you can see the outcome clearly. A very important stepping stone would be to see the outcome as vividly as possible. You have to SEE yourself in that "new" body.

A picture of a famous person or model could help in visualizing what you would want to look like. Who do you admire? Whose body do you find attractive? Put it up on the wall for you to look at.

See yourself in the body you want.

Why not? It may sound stupid at first, but this can be life transforming. Visualizing should be a daily practice. Visualizing and seeing "you" with your desired physical appearance or fitness. Believe me, it works.

The thing that keeps me interested is the shape I can see my body moving into. Strength progression is evident within a few months and the feelings generated in this kind of new found strength are life transforming.

I feel great and I want to continue to feel great.

You need to get a clear picture in your head of what you would like to look like for you to attain these feelings. See yourself with your new body. Feel yourself being as fit as you would like to be. You will be "alive" when this happens. It will be very believable for you with your new eating plan and high energy levels.

HAVE FUN

The idea is to have fun with this. Nothing in this book should be a chore. If you're not having fun with particular exercises or practises, you should not be doing them. The most important feeling here is to feel alive and to have fun.

Visualization and faith is the key to bringing out the success you crave.

LOVE

Love the body you're in. If you don't love yourself, how do you expect yourself to love you back? Sounds cynical right? The key is to start from within and to work your way out.

So you have to start loving your body before any external changes can take place. Ask anyone with a great body if they love themselves. I guarantee you they do.

Chapter 3

TRAIN LIKE A FREAK

This part of the book is all about how far you should push yourself. A lot of the motivation on writing this book and helping people is based around this chapter. I wish that someone could have given me this advice when I was in my teens.

THE MUSCLE IS CAPABLE OF SO MUCH MORE

First you have to understand that "warming up" is absolutely essential. It is almost impossible to tear or injure the muscle when it is properly warm.

There is very little limitation as far as pushing the muscle is concerned.

For you to get the best physical results possible, going a little further, going the extra mile is very important. Never count to ten or twelve or even fifteen in your repetitions.

Always go until you physically fail to complete any more repetitions.

REACHING FAILURE

"Going till failure" might as well have been the title of this book. Three sets or five sets, if you include your warm up, is all you need. Two sets for warm up at half your maximum weight range should be practiced.

WARM UP—2sets at half your usual weight range with 10-12 repetitions each.

So when you can bench press 60 kilograms, AT LEAST half of that should be used as a warm up. It is important to do the warm up slowly and to stretch your muscle WHILE doing the exercise to prevent any injury. Always keep in mind that you are going to put some serious strain on the muscle, so it is important to do a set or two (depending on experience) to prepare your muscle for a serious workout.

When you can feel that your muscle is properly warm, you can advance to training the muscle. Depending on the muscle groups you're targeting, next to follow will be at least 3 sets at maximum effort. 3 sets are sufficient when applied properly.

NOTE; less than a minute is the required rate between the warm up sets and the 3 maximum repetitions.

TRAINING—3 sets (maximum repetitions)

NOTE; you want to gradually increase the weight of the 3 sets.

I'll use the example of a barbell bench press. When you know you can handle 60 kilograms of weight, start with 40 kilograms. If you are doing 8 repetitions and you feel that you are capable of more, and it seems too easy, give it a rest of no more than a minute, adding a bit more weight. This is the testing period for inexperienced athletes. So now you might try 50 kilograms. If the same thing happens and you feel that it is too light, then step it up again.

YOU WANNA GET ATLEAST 3 GREAT SETS.

It only takes one or two repetitions to get the feeling of the weight. It should be heavy enough to reach failure at around 10 repetitions.

Let's say that you are capable of doing 8 repetitions with 50 kilograms.

1st Set—max reps—50kg (max 60kg)

We will regard this as your first set because you are now going to do less than twelve repetitions reaching failure. It is very important that you reach that level of failure.

SPOTTER ESSENTIAL TO AVOID INJURY

So a spotter would come in handy. So we now know that 50 kilograms is a comfortable weight to do the first set.

You absolutely have to push to the last set where you can actually see your arms failing to get the barbell up. That's when your spotter steps in.

So now we will advance to set number two. Let's say you reached 13 repetitions and you succeeded until failure. So now we are going to add some weight and we will be pushing 60 kilograms, which you thought you were capable of handling anyway.

2nd Set—max reps—60kg

Let's say you have been training for a few months and your muscles got used to lifting 60 kilograms. With that you actually surprise yourself by doing 10 repetitions. You should by now feel that your muscle has been under some pressure. You will be tired.

You have to feel tired but strong.

The muscle must at least feel like it is doing some strenuous exercising. Now you will easily be able to advance to 70 kilograms just having done 10 repetitions on 60 kilograms.

Now we are going to reach failure on 70 kilograms and it is important that we are able to do at least 6 repetitions.

You always reach at least 6 repetitions on you're last set.

Weight needs to be adjusted to reach 6 repetitions or as close to that as possible while attempting failure.

3rd set—max reps—70kg

Really push because you know that your muscle is warm and injury is very unlikely. Bear in mind that your muscle is capable of much more than what we think we know or what we have been let to believe.

You're mind is telling you to stop because that's where it normally stops.

YOUR MIND IS NOT TELLING YOU TO STOP

This statement will become evident when you get more comfortable around the weights. You can do another set and add 5kg if it seems plausible for you. Make sure before attempting that you can reach 6 repetitions. Simply give it up if you are struggling to do the first one.

4th set—max reps—75kg

This program varies from muscle group to muscle group, but the basics stay the same. A program is present in this book and other training secrets will be revealed as we go along.

What we are going to talk about next is going to involve the programme and which muscle groups to tackle together. You want to train 4-5 days a week; 3 days weight training if weight loss is required.

So it is best to work out a programme so you don't focus too much on specific areas. It's important not to neglect certain areas. You will start to look out of proportion in several months of training when certain areas are developed and certain areas are standing still.

It is always wise to do legs, or even parts of them, on one day and to really focus on them. Mondays are good for legs because you will or should feel well rested with lots of energy from the weekend. They take the most amount of energy compared to other muscle groups. Therefore a programme should be in place to compliment the muscle group. Legs and lower back work well together. You can mix it up as you go along while you are learning different programs and schedules.

NOTE; it is vital that you mix your schedule so you're muscles don't get used to the same old routine. The same goes for different exercises.

It's up to you to vary muscle groups so they don't get used to the same old boring programme. Arms and shoulders together with traps are a favourite of mine while doing chest and back together to achieve optimum results.

When you are training your back, you are not using your chest, which means you have a perfect muscle ready for work on the same day.

Tearing the muscle for a new layer to grow over and essentially making it stronger, is what we want to achieve. That is what we are doing here, tearing and repairing. To reach maximum levels in tearing, we want to do more exercises involving a specific muscle group.

FOUR EXERCISES INVOLVING THE
SAME MUSCLE GROUP

We'll use the chest as an example. How many chest exercises should we go for? At least four different exercises on the chest muscle group. The best exercises will be reviewed later.

Marcel le Roux

How many upper back exercises should we aim for? At least four should be considered. With shoulders, it is important to really go for gold. Shoulders and legs are the muscle groups that get used all day by most people, so it is more difficult to reach that stretching affect we have been talking about. Four exercises are sufficient for shoulders depending on the intensity level reached by the individual. You can squeeze in a few more sets in an exercise when you feel that you have not been able to push hard enough.

NOTE; drop sets can be considered to reach optimum levels of "stretching".

NOTE; it is important to focus on the muscle while you are "attending" to it. This means that you can't come back to the muscle group within 2 days when resting is required. Therefore focusing on the muscle will work to your advantage.

Train one muscle very well, rather than training them all at once.

The same goes for legs. You use them all day and sometimes mixing programmes can get you the intensity level you'll be looking for. With legs, I often do ten sets of ten repetitions with half the weight I am capable of, then moving on to the next exercise to reach that burn that I'm looking for.

NOTE; the only way you'll be able to tell whether you have done enough, is when you feel that burning sensation.

TEN SETS OF TEN REPETITIONS

What I would like for you to concentrate on is squats when using half the usual weight range you normally lift. If you normally squat 60 kilograms including the weight of the bar, then use half of that.

Remember to work out what the bar weighs. The bar can weigh up to 20 kilograms on its own. We are going to do ten sets with ten repetitions each. You should start out pretty comfortable. The intensity should progress while the big muscle himself is getting completely warmed up. It is also not necessary to follow a warm up session in this exercise. It is, however, important that you don't allow more than a minute in between sets.

If there are two sets left and you feel that you haven't reached a higher intensity level than usual, then gradually increase the weight. This can be done on the last two sets.

IMPORTANT; DO NOT rest longer than a minute in between sets or repetitions in any exercise you attempt. Take a sip of water during that minute. Take a couple of deep breaths before continuing.

USE THE CLOCK

You can rest after a muscle group has been targeted. Plan out what you will target for the day. Get your exercises ready in your head or on paper so confusion or hesitation can be avoided. You need to know what you will be attempting depending on your level of experience. When you have finished a set, grab a sip of water and get ready for the next. After the exercise is completed, hurry on to the next within the minute and start targeting the same muscle group. Do four exercises.

You can rest for up to 5 minutes after the muscle group has been targeted. Your heart will be racing and you will feel pumped ready for the next exercise.

GO HOME

What do you do if you don't feel like you hold any power or have enough energy to reach failure? You simply walk out the door; get into your car and go home. Go home and start preparing for the next day. It is as simple as that.

Even if you've only been in the gym for twenty minutes, turn around and stop wasting your time. Nothing is going to change.

You are NOT going to start feeling great if you continue to train.

Go home and stack up on the good stuff. Take your vitamins, prepare yourself a balanced meal and take a protein shake before you go to bed together with a fruit. Make sure you do the same the next day starting in the morning with energy rich foods every 2-3 hours. That will get you going.

Chapter 4

SUPLEMENTS

Supplements can play a very important part in your training and fitness. I'm going to discuss things like protein shakes and creatine. There are a lot of these products on the market introduced by many different companies. Companies work on profit, so they will put a lot of products out there that you think you need. Many of them can be use full and many of them won't be necessary for developments in your energy levels. Some of them, however, play a crucial role in attaining results. I'll only talk about the ones that can change the way you think about supplements.

PROTEIN SHAKES

Protein is the basic building material for muscle tissue. Strength trainers need to consume more than the average daily allowance. Protein intake should not exceed 2 grams per kilogram of bodyweight. Half that may even be adequate for developments, depending on level of fitness.

Protein shakes vary. They are very simple to understand though. It will only take a glance at the back of the container to find out what it consists of. That is important because YOU will be consuming those ingredients.

How much protein do we aim for? 2grams of protein per kilogram of bodyweight should be your target. Remember that protein that we don't use also turn into fat. Protein also expands the fat cells in the body. So we want to get to 2g per kilogram or as close to that as possible. You are still recovering on non training days, so you want to at least get half of your desired protein intake.

EXAMPLE; your weight is 80 kilograms—you are taking 80g of carbohydrates and 160 g of protein. Getting as close to that will be very beneficial to reach maximum energy levels and increase recovery time.

NOTE; these figures should be used as indicators only. Consumption should depend on your strength and fitness and over all energy levels.

Protein shakes with little or no carbohydrates work best because of the 1g of carbohydrate per kilogram of body weight rule. If the protein shake contains any or too much carbohydrates, then you are going to over shoot the carbohydrate rule by at least twice the amount.

EXAMPLE; if you are taking 30g of carbohydrates per shake and consuming a couple of shakes in a day, and you only weigh 60 kilograms, then you can clearly see that our target is not anywhere near our 1g rule.

30g + 30g = 60g of carbohydrates

If you count in all the other carbohydrates that you include in the foods consumed, then you will surely at least double the 1g rule.

NOTE; it is recommended that you take in enough carbohydrates to reach energy levels desired. The best option would be to select a whey product that does not contain the carbohydrates you want to avoid. I'd rather eat an apple than some protein shake carbohydrates.

FAT

Fat is an essential nutrient, however, you require a small amount to maintain that much needed energy levels during exercise. Less than 30 % of your calorie intake should come from unsaturated fat.

CARBOHYDRATES

A large number of carbohydrate calories are needed to fuel both workouts and tissue building. While getting enough calories is important, it is also important to get the right kind of calories.

Carbohydrates are the predominant energy source for strength training. The harder you work out the more carbohydrates you will need.

My recommended allowance would be 1 gram per kilogram of bodyweight. However, that rule can easily be overshot depending on the level of physicality achieved.

Energy should be stored every 2-3 hours with the hope of completing strenuous exercises.

Carbohydrates you don't use turn into fat and then make you look bigger. That's the illusion.

You are not stronger and fitter. So look for a lean protein or whey protein. I would not do more than 2 shakes a day or a maximum of 3, if you decide to take one before going to bed. Remember that protein is part of the fuel for the muscle when it is recovering. Your muscle is recovering when you sleep. So taking it before going to bed is a very wise decision.

How many carbohydrates do we aim for? 1gram of carbohydrates per kilogram of bodyweight should be your target. Remember that carbohydrates that we don't use also turn into fat. So we want to get to 1g per kilogram or as close to that as possible. You are still recovering on non training days, so you want to at least get half of your desired carbohydrate intake.

NOTE; it can be easy to exceed the amount on strenuous training.

EXAMPLE; your weight is 80 kilograms—you are taking 80g of carbohydrates and 160 g of protein. Getting as close to that will be very beneficial to reach maximum energy levels and increase recovery time.

NOTE; these figures should be used as indicators only. Consumption should depend on your strength and fitness and over all energy levels.

CREATINE

Creatine occurs naturally in the body and helps to supply energy to the muscles. It is transported in the blood for use by muscles. Approximately half of stored creatine in the body originates from food with meat being the best dietary source of creatine. Vegetables do not contain creatine; as a result, lower levels of muscle creatine are present in vegetarians.

Creatine supplements are used by athletes to gain muscle mass. It effectively improves the response to resistance exercises, increasing the production of muscles. I don't train without it and my advice would be to do the same. I do however use the resting period where creatine is not consumed. Alcohol should be avoided and lots of water should be consumed especially during training.

NOTE; creatine supplementation can also be replaced by a higher protein diet.

NOTE; taking more than the usual dosage of creatine offers no added benefit.

There are different types of creatine and new developments are available on the market every year. Magazines tend to help in soughing out these new developments. The market is getting bigger and bigger for new emerging products to become available. In our modern world studies have grown significantly to create "bigger" and better products. I will reveal my favourite in the next segment.

NITRIC OXIDE

There are a variety of products on the market that contains nitric oxide. This helps with distribution of nutrients inside the muscle and improves the uptake by the cell. Products that are out there like NO-explode, dramatically enhances the workout therefore contributing to an intense workout. It reduces lactic acid build up, replenishes lost electrolytes, and saturates the muscle with nutrients necessary for growth. I highly recommend experimenting with new products.

Products like NO-Xplode provide you with enough energy and confidence to be a few steps ahead in physical development.

THE BOTTOM LINE IS THAT YOU ARE GUARANTEED A GREAT WORKOUT.

When it comes to other products, you will need to stay on top of things by trying different products and reading up on them to see if they're really worth it. You don't want to spend your whole salary on supplements.

NOTE; consult a registered nutritionist, physician or other health care provider for personal nutritional counselling. This information is not intended as a substitute for appropriate medical treatment.

Chapter 5

CARDIO

Cardio should follow after weight training and NOT before weight training. It takes a lot from the body to reach failure and I want to use the maximum amount of energy in doing all I can in the weight lifting department; this way you will ease into cardio exercises with greater energy levels.

I on the other hand, don't have any weight to lose and can almost consume anything I want without storing any fat. Now some people are not that fortunate and should follow a slightly different plan. Both plans will be discussed and should also be understood by individuals who don't need to lose weight.

STICK TO THIS PLAN FOR OPTIMUM RESULTS

Follow below example if you would like to lose more weight or if your energy levels aren't as high as it could be. This program can increase the knowledge of individuals who wish not to lose much weight. This will develop a much needed understanding between weightlifting and cardio.

Marcel le Roux

I do very little cardio, and if I do, a simple ten minute run is enough for me. This follows after weight training, when there is still enough gas left in the tank. I usually only attempt this for fun.

NOTE; when attempting any cardio, only stay in the gym for as long as you feel great.

You can feel tired, you must feel tired, but you shouldn't feel like you want to pass out. You might have taken it a little too far and need to work on getting your energy levels on maximum.

If you reach the point where you are drained and hesitant on attempting any cardio, then simply turn around and go home. Start preparing for the next day so that you do have the energy to focus on cardio.

A few minutes for water consumption can also be taken to asses your level of fatigue.

Dehydration also needs to be treated when symptoms develop. A chapter has been included in the latter part of the book.

Do the form of cardio that you enjoy. If it isn't fun then don't do it.

LOSING WEIGHT

You are still going to concentrate on weight lifting by following your programme and therefore easing into cardio exercises. This is a great way of "coming alive" in the gym. This will give you the motivation for getting into cardio.

MAXIMUM ENERGY LEVELS NEED TO BE REACHED

This is the quickest and most fun way of losing weight.

High energy levels need to be reached for you to perform well enough to lose weight.

Enjoyment in doing something is where results are showing.

Results, together with feeling great, is the goal.

A focus on weight training for the first couple of weeks is essential.

Only minimum amounts of cardio can be exercised. Running for as long as you can without walking would also be essential in the first two weeks.

A gradual increase in energy will be evident in the following two weeks. Weight loss will also start on a rapid rate during weeks 4-6.

|W   6

|E

|I   5

|G

|H   4

|T

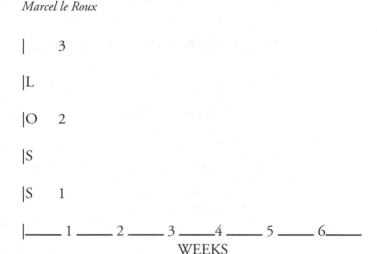

```
|     3

|L

|O   2

|S

|S   1

|____ 1 ____ 2 ____ 3 ____ 4 ____ 5 ____ 6____
```
                            WEEKS

This is when you will start to feel more comfortable while your body is adapting to the exercise.

20-30 MINUTES CARDIO

Weight lifting is thus followed by cardio. I would suggest to do 20-30 minutes (20 minutes if your energy levels are very low) of weight training concentrating on reaching failure. Remember the warm up stage consisting of 2 sets at half your maximum range. Do 12 repetitions of each.

Make sure you can feel the muscle stretching while you are doing the weight lifting. This is a pleasant feeling.

Only focus on one muscle group per day when weight loss is a part of your target.

Another focus must be the main muscle groups that will be most beneficial for strength and weight loss. Concentrate only on these exercises. They are the most important for beginners alike. Here is a list of these exercises.

- DEAD LIFTS
- BARBELL SQUATS
- BARBELL BENCH PRESS

The odd exercise can be added when energy levels start to increase.

The above exercises are the most important and should be taken seriously whenever attempting.

Please be advised by your local personal trainer in reaching a level of optimum technique and correct stance.

These correct techniques are vital in targeting the muscle and are absolutely necessary. Otherwise, you would be standing there all day only to be trying to target those muscles that are so important.

These exercises should go on till reaching failure and should be attempted on individual days. Maximum amounts of repetitions should be exercised while attempting.

Day 1—DEAD LIFTS
Day 2—BARBELL SQUATS
Day 3—BARBELL BENCH PRESS

4-5 DAYS TRAINING

The programme can simply be started again during the same week, given the fact that you have already rested the muscle for 2 days. That is if you are training 4-5 days a week.

On each day exercises should be combined with exercises involving the main muscle groups you are focusing on in your 20-30 minute gap. That means that you could bring in other exercises to in affect increase strain on the same muscle. You will be targeting a muscle group for the whole 20-30 minutes. Make sure that a minute is not exceeded during sets or during repetitions.

NOTE; 20-30 minutes weight training and 20-30 minutes cardio apply.

So on day one you will be doing dead lifts together with other exercises that target the same muscle group. Hamstrings and lower back can be done on the same day. I have included the best targeting exercises in my programmes. There are great exercises you can follow, depending on the facilities available to you. Personal trainers will be able to assist in finding and guiding you to suitable exercises.

Have a rest before you move on to the cardio exercises. Another 20-30 minutes of cardio will do. Give yourself a couple of weeks to ease into maximum energy levels if you find it difficult to do this much exercise at full pace.

GIVE AS MUCH EFFORT DURING THE EXERCISE.

IF THAT MEANS THAT YOUR TIME SPENT IN THE
GYM IS VERY LIMITING, THEN SO BE IT.

You WILL start feeling great when the right fuel is
being filled up.

Energy levels will be lower in an overweight individual
than in someone that is in perfect weight. That is normal
and will slowly start to change if you STICK TO THE
PROGRAMME.

Extensive details are included in the training programmes
section of the book.

Chapter 6

DEHYDRATION

Dehydration is defined as an excessive loss of body fluid. It is literally the removal of water. Symptoms may include headaches similar to what is experienced during a hangover.

LOSS OF PERFORMANCE OF UP TO 30%

Experiences of low endurance, rapid heart rates, high body temperatures and fatigue are some of the things we want to avoid during training. Water as a result, then becomes a huge part of nutrition.

Dehydration is best avoided by drinking sufficient amounts of water. The greater the amount of water lost through perspiration, the greater the amount of water consumed as a replacement to avoid dehydration.

During exercise, relying on thirst alone may be insufficient to prevent dehydration.

When urine is lightly coloured or colourless, chances are that dehydration is not occurring.

A full bladder must then be developed at least every 3-5 hours. When you are doing strenuous exercises, a full bladder can be experienced in little time. Regular sips of water should therefore be consumed. Water intake will not be adequate to maintain proper hydration when urine is deeply coloured or when urination does not occur.

Water loss can increase through perspiration during warm or humid environments or during strenuous exercise. Losses of water in a person's body during an average day in temperature (even in much colder countries), can be anything around 2 litres of water.

Drinking water beyond the needs of the body entails little risk when done in moderation, since the kidneys will efficiently remove any excess water through the urine.

TAKE REGULAR SIPS OF WATER—ESPECIALLY DURING TRAINING SESSIONS

Chapter 7

EATING PROGRAMMES

MEAL 1 BREAKFAST

OPTION 1

Half a cup of cooked oats OR oat bran with one scoop of pure protein (half a serving).
I cup of tea with skimmed milk.
1 green apple OR half a grape fruit.

OPTION 2

One slice of seed loaf OR rye bread
Two egg whites and one whole egg.
One cup of tea.
One pear OR one peach.

Option 3

One grilled fish fillet
Half a cup of bran flakes
One cup of tea

Two plums OR half a grapefruit

NOTE; water should be consumed during the day and not during meals.

MEAL 2—MID MORNING

One serving of whey protein.

NOTE; a fruit can be consumed during this time if it hasn't been included in Meal 1.

MEAL 3—LUNCH

OPTION 1

One sweet potato OR potato (baked or micro waved).
One skinless chicken breast or fish fillet (micro waved or grilled)
One cup of cooked broccoli.

OPTION 2

One slice of seed loaf of rye bread.
One tin of tuna in spring water.
One green apple or two slices of pineapple.
Half a cup of mixed vegetables.

OPTION 3

Lean beef minced meat with tomato.
Half a cup of pasta.
1 cup of salad with lemon juice and olive oil.

NOTE; these meals are going to be 2-3 hours apart. Remember to take water in between those times. Allow 30 minutes before and after meals.

MEAL 4 MID AFTERNOON

One serving of whey protein.

NOTE; a half a serving can also be consumed depending on training schedule and intensity level achieved during training sessions.

MEAL 5—DINNER

OPTION 1

One skinless chicken breast or hake fillet. 2 cups of cooked broccoli or stir fry vegetables.

OPTION 2

One tin of solid tune in spring water or tune salad. Use only light mayonnaise.
One cup of mixed vegetables.

OPTION 3

One lean grilled steak.
One cup of steamed green beans OR peas with carrots.

MEAL 6

One serving of whey protein (half a serving may also be adequate).

NOTE; meal 6 is optional. No meals to be consumed after 8 pm.

NOTE; chicken, fish or steak can be measured to about 150 grams.

Chapter 8

TRAINING SCEDULES

Herein is some examples of advanced training schedules designed to get you to perform to you maximum levels of output by reaching FAILURE.

We want to reach failure in every repetition that we attempt.

This programme will include a cardio run of no more than 10 minutes a day after weight training. It will only be recommended on days when you feel you have enough energy left. Running can also be included in days where you aren't doing any weight training when excess weight needs to be shed.

NOTE; it is important to focus on weight training to get energy levels up. This is how you will be able to focus on cardio with ease once you have reached that level of success.

That means that you can leave cardio out of your programme for the first two weeks, depending on the amount of weight that needs to be shed. This will make it easier, physically and mentally to attempt cardio exercises after a success period of up to 4 weeks.

Monday or day1—CHEST AND BACK

Tuesday or day 2—LEGS AND LOWER BACK

Wednesday or day 3—SHOULDERS AND ARMS

Thursday or day 1—CHEST AND BACK

Friday or day 2—LEGS AND LOWER BACK

The program stays the same whether you resting on Wednesdays, Fridays or Saturdays.

You are squeezing in all the muscle groups in on 3 days. You start again with the same programme after your 3 days regardless of what day it is. If you start with doing chest on a Monday, give it two days until you attempt training on the muscle group again.

NOTE; rather have an off day than a day where you aren't training to your full potential. Aim to reach failure.

Intermediate (weight loss)

Monday or day 1—CHEST

Tuesday or day 2—BACK AND BICEPS

Wednesday or day 3—LEGS AND CALVES

Thursday or day 4—SHOULDERS AND TRICEPS

Friday or day 5—HAMSTRINGS AND LOWER

BACK

What happens when you miss a day? You simply do what you were supposed to do on the next training day.

NOTE; abdominal muscles were left out for you to decide on which days you prefer to include abdominal exercises.

The fact is that we all possess six pack abdominals; they are just hidden underneath the fat. The first thing you need to do is to target the cardio exercises before you can focus on the abdominals. It's easier and more beneficial to target certain areas first.

You will spend all your energy on one area to make sure you're really targeting the area.

There's less use in doing everything at once. That is one of the reasons why most people don't achieve results in months of training.

On the intermediate or weight loss programme we want to do no less than 20 minutes of cardio exercises after weight training. You want to this virtually every day.

IMPORTANT CARDIO TIPS

When running is not a part of your cardio programmes, a minimum of 30 minutes will be required. A minimum of 20 minutes is required when you are including running (10 minutes) in your programme.

20 minutes of cardio that includes 10 minutes of running

Or

30 minutes of cardio that doesn't include running

RUNNING IS THE ULTIMATE CARDIO EXERCISE

5 minutes of running will soon turn into 15 minutes of running when you're energy levels are on a certain level. It's not the easiest thing to do for most people, because of the muscles that are being used, that of which are not yet developed.

-It may take up to 4 weeks to adapt; regardless of any excess weight.

You're lungs also need to get used to the amount of oxygen you body is demanding. All these developments need to be accounted for.

Once the muscles get developed AND energy levels are running high AND you're lungs have adapted, only then WILL you be running for 15 minutes with ease.

That is the only way people are capable of running marathons while you are sitting there asking yourself how "they" are capable of that amount of running. By jolly they must be special.

NOTE; it is important that you feel good while doing whatever cardio it is you're doing.

You are however going to be out of breath and possibly be really tired.

NOTE; the further you push yourself today, the easier it will be the next week. The quicker you will get yourself to the level of required development needed to "accomplish" fitness.

There should not be a feeling of hunger together with tiredness. Enough energy is needed while attempting any exercise.

NOTE; stop with whatever cardio it is you are doing if you have a dry throat. Take two minutes or more and stack up on water.

TAKE IN WATER WHILE ATTEMPTING ANY TRAINING

Exercises I recommend that provide the ultimate results.

BARBBELL BENCH PRESS

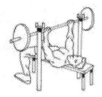

INCLINE DUMBBELL CHEST PRESS

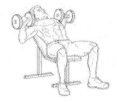

DUMBBELL CHEST FLY

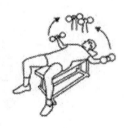

PULL OVERS

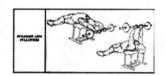

WIDE GRIP PULL UPS

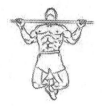

BENT OVER ROW

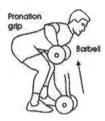

SHRUGS

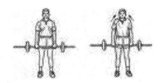

REVERSE FLY

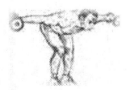

DUMBBELL/ BARBELL SHOULDER PRESS

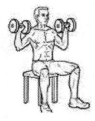

UPRIGHT ROW

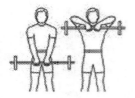

LATERAL RAISE

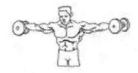

BENT OVER LATERAL RAISE

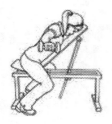

OVERHEAD EXTENSIONS

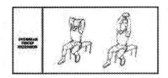

TRICEP DIPS

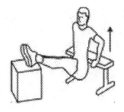

TRICEP KICKBACKS

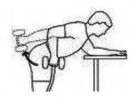

TRICEP SCULLCRUSHERS

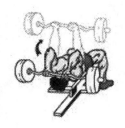

DEADLIFTS

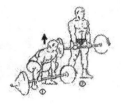

LEG PRESS

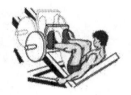

SQUATS

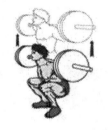

LEG EXTENSION

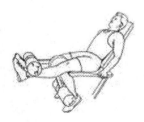

Marcel le Roux

BARBBELL CURLS

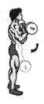

HAMMER CURLS

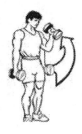

CONSENTRATION CURLS

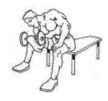

PREACHER CURLS

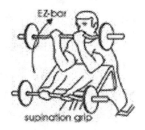

These exercises are the most important and most effective for targeting muscle groups and should be attempted first. If you feel that you are able to do any more exercises, then by jolly, please do so.

TRAINING PROGRAMMES

INTERMEDIATE TO ADVANCE

An example of a 3 day exercise programme will be discussed in further detail.

NOTE; the same programme will be presented to intermediate and advanced candidates. Intermediates should train 3 times a week using this program while 4-5 days can be followed for advanced candidates. Simply start the 3 day cycle in the same week starting at day 1.

This could be one of the most enjoyable parts of attaining one's desired physique.

NOTE; this part should be taken seriously and NOT be neglected.

On day 1 you will start with chest and back.

On day 2 you will start with legs and lower back.

On day 3 you will start with shoulders and arms.

Marcel le Roux

DAY 1

BARBBELL BENCH PRESS
INCLINE DUMBBELL CHEST PRESS
DUMBBELL CHEST FLY
PULL OVERS

WIDE GRIP PULL UPS
BENT OVER ROW
SHRUGS
REVERSE FLY

DAY 2

SEATED CALVE RAISES
CALVE PRESS

DEADLIFTS
LEG PRESS
SQUATS
LEG EXTENSION
HAMSTRING EXTENSIONS

DAY 3

DUMBBELL/ BARBELL SHOULDER PRESS
UPRIGHT ROW
LATERAL RAISE
BENT OVER LATERAL RAISE

OVERHEAD EXTENSIONS
TRICEP DIPS
TRICEP KICKBACKS

TRICEP SCULLCRUSHERS

BARBBELL CURLS
HAMMER CURLS
CONSENTRATION CURLS
PREACHER CURLS

It is important to complete as many of these exercises as possible. They are combined together to guarantee optimum results. I did NOT just throw them in there to fill these pages. They work well together. Failure should be reached as often as possible or whenever the body allows it.

A TRAINING PARTNER CAN BE VERY BENEFICIAL IN MOTIVATION AND IN WITNESSING FAILURE.

TEN SETS OF TEN

10 sets of 10 repetitions should be followed every second week on particular exercises. Here is a list of these exercises.

LATERAL BENCH PRESS
SQUATS
DEADLIFTS

You are doing squats and dead lifts on the same day, therefore to alternate squats and dead lifts would be wise. Energy will run out when attempting these together especially applying 10 sets of 10 repetitions.

Remember to use half the weight that you usually use when attempting 10 sets. That means; if you are pressing 50 kilograms (including the bar), then 25 kilograms should be used (when attempting 10 sets).

WARM UP

The warm up will depend on which muscle group you are targeting. Work on this example until you start to learn the adequate warm up sensation. Do two sets at half the maximum weight range you normally succeed in. Make sure you stretch the muscle while doing this exercise. Do 12 repetitions.

NOTE; only two sets need to be completed before you're training session commences. The warm up targets the whole muscle group.

PUMPING IRON

This is where the fun begins. You want to do at least 3 sets on each individual exercise.

NOTE; a fourth set can be added after 2 months of experience on this programme. This will give you time to get to know yourself working with the program.

FAILURE, FAILURE, FAILURE ON EACH SET

Here is an example of the weight range that should be followed.

We want to pick three different weight ranges before commencing on each individual set. We want to gradually increase the weight. For example; 30-40-45 kilograms;

20-23-25 kilograms. Simply add more weight to do a fourth set.

We want to effectively reach failure in all 3 sets NOT exceeding 12 repetitions. You also want to do at least 6 repetitions on the last set.

DO THE EXERCISE SLOWLY

The muscle should be stretching while exercising. You want to feel the muscle. It should be warm to be able to experience this stretchy feeling. This is vital when you want to see results. You also need to be in control of the weights. This is the part where nutrition will play a crucial role.

ONE MINUTE REST IN BETWEEN SETS

No more than a minute should be allowed in between sets. You're muscle start to cool down after a minute. You need to target them while they are still warm. Water needs to be consumed during that minute.

TECHNNIQUE

Always keep the back straight when attempting any exercise. Personal trainers usually know how to apply the correct technique. They can be helpful when a certain exercise requires a spotter. Please make use of them.

IMPORTANT; on the first and second day (particularly on the second day) when muscles are recovering, a recovering muscle "pain" should be felt. When you experience that burning sensation, and only then, have you experienced true muscle building. Maximum strength and fitness will be evident within 2 months. More weight will be lifted due to the "pain" induced on the muscle. YOU WILL FEEL GREAT.

BEGINNERS

Beginners are going to follow a slightly different plan.

It doesn't mean that are a beginner or an elderly person, that you are not capable of strength building. You are.

Monday or day 1—CHEST

Tuesday or day 2—BACK AND BICEPS

Wednesday or day 3—LEGS AND CALVES

Thursday or day 4—SHOULDERS AND TRICEPS

Friday or day 5—HAMSTRINGS AND LOWER

BACK

It is important to warm up and to do the exercise slowly. Still go for that stretching affect. It is NOT something only professional's attempt. Everyone should be practicing this.

Listen to your body when joint pains are experienced. This could be due to pressure on the joints or due to undeveloped muscle. Give the muscle enough resting time. Ease in to it. There is no rush. It can take weeks for your body to adapt depending on fitness levels. You should however start feeling comfortable within a few weeks.

NOTE; do not attempt when pains are severe. Consult your physician.

Warm-up will also consist of two sets for beginners.

-2-3 sets of weight training

-a minimum of 20 minutes on weights

-a minimum of 20 minutes on cardio

Everything else applies to everyone. Woman, old, young, strong, everyone. Play with these exercises and start to feel great. Anyone that is in excellent shape, are using some or all of these techniques. You too can attain that of which is truly yours. Enjoy.